Methadone, What Every Family Should Know

Prologue

As a substance abuse counselor in a methadone clinic I've worked with hundreds of opiate addicts; many who've succeeded in their treatment and many who have not. It has been my experience that many leave too early from treatment for numerous reasons. My purpose for writing this is to help those who are searching for a pathway out of the world of street drugs. It is also my hope, that this material will help those currently in methadone treatment learn more about it.

I will be referring to methadone treatment throughout this book; however this author recognizes Buprenorphine treatment as an equally valid treatment option. Buprenorphine is the active ingredient in Suboxone ® and Subutex ®. These drugs have some advantages and some disadvantages as compared to methadone; however this is beyond the scope of this book.

Should you or anyone you care about enter into opiate replacement therapy (methadone treatment), please inquire as to whether methadone or Buprenorphine will be your best choice. Rely on the counselors and the medical staff of your clinic to advise you.

Getting Started

When chemically dependent people decide they want help, they've come to a place in life where they realize they can no longer survive in their drug addicted lifestyle. Those who turn to methadone treatment for help are usually exhausted, have lost friends, family, jobs, and financial assets and are on the brink of losing even more.

As a substance abuse counselor in a methadone clinic, I find that very few enter treatment on the order of the court. Most patients enter treatment on their own; however they may be directed to do so by their spouse, significant other, or a parent. I have learned that walking through the front door of a treatment center takes a lot of courage, yet in many ways, choosing treatment is also an act of desperation.

When an opiate dependent person enters treatment, they typically don't know what else to do or where else to turn. But, they have learned, usually the hard way that more drug use will only lead to more losses. Drug addicts are usually tired of the stealing, lying, cheating, scamming, and all the other deviant behaviors that drug addicts are known for. I hear stories every day, and as soon as I think I've heard the most outrageous story, I hear a new one.

If you've bought this book for yourself, or you've bought it for someone else, chances are you have your own stories to tell. Here are two short stories I've come across:

1) There's the story of Gene who got high on Xanax's before he got onto opiates. He told me about the time his aunt came by to visit his family from out of town. He told me

that while the family was visiting in the living room, he stole his aunt's purse and went into his bedroom where he stole all her pills and took her car keys. Then he said that he quietly walked out the back door and drove his aunt's car to the beer store. He told me that he blacked out for moment and ended up in the woods. When he woke up the car was stuck in the mud. He said he revved up the engine and the tires would spin in the leaves and the mud creating a lot of smoke. He couldn't get any traction and he continued the rev up the engine. He kept gunning the motor faster until the leaves caught on fire. Eventually the car was engulfed in flames and he had to exit the vehicle once it filled with smoke. The car burst into flames and burnt up entirely. The tires burnt up, the seats burnt up, the carpet burnt up, all the rubber hoses and belts burnt up, and even some of the metal parts of the car were warped or melted. The car was total loss. As he sat in my office and as he finished his story he hung his head and said, "How can I say I'm sorry for that?" I said, "Well you just have to try." But I am perplexed that even with a story like this; he was not willing to seek treatment at that time.
2) I had one patient tell me about his sister who came home and found their mother dead on the couch. The sister took her mother's credit cards and maxed them out on a crack and heroin binge. Three days later she came back home and called 911. Obviously, sister didn't want to share the money on the credit card with her siblings. After that, sister still wasn't ready to enter treatment.

It's hard to predict when an addict will finally say enough is enough and choose to enter treatment. However, when they do seek treatment, if their drug of choice is Heroin, Oxycontine, Dilaudid, Roxycodone, Hydrocodone, Percocet, Morphine, Fentanyl, and other opiate/opioid based medications, then methadone treatment is an option.

When a opiate addicted person walks into a methadone clinic for treatment, the first thing that's suppose to happen, is that person is "screened." During the screening process a person's drug of choice is determine, plus how long they've been using their drug of choice, how much they use, how much money they spend each day on their drug habit, and how they take their drug (orally, snorting, smoking, injections, etc). From this information a judgment is made as to whether an addict is appropriate for treatment at a methadone clinic.

In truth, methadone treatment works for some but not for others. If a person says they're addicted to crack, cocaine, alcohol, bath salts, marijuana, ecstasy, meth amphetamines, and other drug types then they are *not* appropriate for methadone treatment. Methadone is only suitable for treating opiate addiction.

Another factor as to why methadone works for some and not for others is the fact that most opiate addicts have never taken the time to read about methadone treatment. All that most addicts know about methadone is what they've heard on the street.

I've had several new patients shake my hand, sit down in my office, and say "I'm just going to be here a week or two." Obviously, they have no idea what methadone treatment is all about. As you will learn, methadone treatment takes a year or two, or three, or a life time in many cases to enable an opiate addicted patient to manage his/her addiction, re-enter the straight world, and become productive again. Once they learn that methadone treatment is not a quick fix, they often quit treatment after a few days only to relapse back into the soup of a drug centered lifestyle.

Many new patients suffer from what I call "male pattern thinking." I too have suffered from this type of thinking. Males are often loaners, self reliant, mechanical, and problem solvers. As such, they enter treatment with their own idea as to how they are going to engineer their own recovery.

They get it in their head that addiction is a problem and with methadone they will apply strong will power and overcome their addiction in 7 to 14 days. Problem solved. Unfortunately, *methadone treatment is a treatment not a cure*. And, methadone only works when you take it. The day you stop taking it, is the day it's no longer helping you. After a week or two many get frustrated that their plan didn't work so they give up and go back into the soup. Their problem is that their expectations were unrealistic.

I have had several female clients come into treatment with their boyfriend. After a few days they come back and say their boyfriend is no longer with them. The problem is that boyfriend number 1 said he was going to pay for her methadone treatment, and now that he's gone she has to find another way to pay for treatment. This often means finding a job. Many drug addicts are not prepared to enter the workforce, as they often don't have transportation, housing, or the money to pay for gas, food, and treatment. For some new patient's it doesn't' take long and they fall back into the soup for financial reasons.

Many drug users are also drug dealers. Those who buy drugs always try to make the best deal they can, and often times they come across opportunities to make a few dollars and support their habit as well. Many work as full time dealers to support their own drug use. When a drug dealer enters treatment, they often have to give up their source of income. They find themselves having to pay for daily doses of methadone, but don't have a legitimate job to support their treatment.

I have had several married couples enter treatment who live 45 minutes or an hour away from the clinic. The cost of gas everyday is prohibitive enough, but when you add in the cost of methadone it becomes well over a $1000 a month for a couple. However, $1000 a month is not as much as a $200 per day habit. You do the math. Nonetheless, it's a lot of money for people who have children, and need a car, and a job, and have to live with Mom and Dad who now pay for everything and expect methadone treatment to solve all their problems in 2 or 3 weeks.

The Wayward Captain

I think of opiate addiction as being like a rogue captain sailing wildly out in the sea (the sea of life I suppose). The captain is reckless, and doesn't pay attention to the signs of a shallow reef, and manages to sail into the reef, tearing a hole in the side of his boat. It is at this time the captain wishes to get back to port and give up his/her wild sailing ways. The problem of course is that his ship is taking on water and sinking. The captain has only partial control of his/her boat and he/she cannot guide the boat back to port. As the boat takes on more water the boat is sinking. However, methadone is a lot like tar and other ship repairing materials (at least in this story – in real life methadone is a watery liquid and not like tar). The tar (methadone) along with the right tools (counseling) can be used to repair the hole. Once the hole is repaired, the ship will no longer be taking in water, thus enabling the captain to gain control of the ship and sail it back to port, where he/she can start his/her life again on dry land.

Other treatment options offer good tools like counseling, but they do not address the fact that there is a hole in the ship. The hole is analogous to an opiate dependent brain. Without addressing the day to day dependency, which presents itself in the form of cravings and withdrawal symptoms, the captain is going to try and sail the ship with a big hole in it, and will undoubtedly take on water making it harder to sail hour by hour. As the hole gets larger, such a ship might sink before it even gets close to port.

Many Who Are Chemically Dependent on Opiates Also Have Other Mental Health Problems And Often Reject Methadone Treatment

In the world of substance abuse treatment, many times we come across individuals who are not only diagnosed with opiate abuse disorder, but also have co-occurring mental health issues as well.

Many of these issues are diagnosed by mental health professionals and psychiatrists. Common co-occurring disorders include anxiety, depression, bi-polar, manic depressive, panic attacks, agoraphobia, various behavior disorders, and obsessive compulsive disorder. There are of course many other diagnoses.

Our job as substance abuse counselors is to recognize other mental health diagnosis when they present themselves. It is not the job of a substance abuse counselor to diagnose such disorders, and usually they do not have the expertise or the qualifications to make such a diagnosis. A diagnosis usually comes from a licensed mental health professional or a medical doctor who specializes in behavioral health. Doctors will often prescribe medications to help patients manage their disorder. Common prescriptions include benzodiazepines for anxiety,

PTSD (Post Traumatic Stress Disorder), and panic disorders. Amphetamines are often prescribed for (ADD) Attention Deficit Disorder or (ADHD) Attention Deficit Hyperactivity Disorder.

Common benzodiazepines include: Ativan, Klonopin, Xanax, and Valium

Common amphetamines include: Adderall and Ritalin

Both of the above drug classifications are addictive and can negatively interact with methadone. For this reason these drugs must be coordinated between the methadone clinic and the prescribing doctor. Many methadone clinics have a zero tolerance policy towards benzo's. If they find benzo's in a patient's urine screen that patient is soon removed from the program. Other clinics however are more tolerant of the benzo's, although as mentioned before there must be a coordination of care between the benzo doctor and the methadone doctor. The same is true with amphetamines.

Patients, who have a legitimate prescription from a doctor for benzo's or amphetamines, often find themselves in conflict with their methadone clinic if they choose *not* to coordinate care. This often leaves a client having to choose between staying with methadone treatment, or abandoning it for their other prescription drugs.

Many drug abusers with co-occurring disorders will often hide behind their co-occurring disorder as a reason not to engage in substance abuse treatment. They will often say, "Why should go to a methadone clinic, they won't help me with my bipolar problem?" This excuse somehow allows them to justify their continued use of illicit drugs.

A good clinic however, will work with those who have co-occurring disorders and will help a dual diagnosed patient find a suitable psychiatrist, or behavioral doctor, while the patient remains involved in methadone treatment.

Pain Clinics versus Methadone Clinics

Many people are prescribed pain pills (opiate based pills) for pain. Over time, their daily intake of prescription pain pills increases, or the patient takes more pills than is actually prescribed by their doctor, in an effort to try and better manage their pain. The need for increased drug use is known as "tolerance." Over time a patient's tolerance for pain pills can become so high (high tolerance) that a patient can reach the potential for an overdose. High drug tolerance and heavy drug use is a sign of chemical dependency.

Regardless of how people get addicted to pain pills, many times a methadone clinic is a good choice to get off pills (and heroin). Methadone clinics however do not tolerate pain pill usage. Once a methadone clinic does a prescription drug search, and finds that a patient is being prescribed pain pills from a doctor, the patient is given a choice. The patient can choose to remain in methadone treatment while terminating their opiate prescription, or they can choose to terminate their methadone treatment and stay with their opiate prescribing doctor. A patient cannot play both sides of the fence however. In some clinics this decision is required immediately, once the pain pill prescription has been discovered. After all methadone clinics treat opiate addiction, they are not a pain clinic. And if you think about it, being treated for opiate addiction while having a prescription for opiates is not a very good recovery plan.

Many patients over time bounce back and forth between the use of opiates from a pain doctor and the methadone center. Once the pain doctor discovers that the patient is on methadone the pain doctor discontinues the prescription of opiate based pain pills in order for the pain doctor to preserves his/her license to practice. When the methadone clinic does a prescription drug search and finds that the patient is taking opiates from a pain doctor, the client is given a choice to either terminate their use of methadone or terminate their use of opiate based pain pills. Many patients who live in a smaller metropolitan area find that there is a limited number of pain doctors and methadone clinics from which to choose from. As a result they can burn their bridges in their local area and find themselves stuck without professional help. Such a client will often turn to street opiates usually leading to uncontrolled usage.

There does appear to be a need for a 3rd type of treatment facility. Since a pain doctor cannot legally prescribe an opiate to a methadone patient, and since a methadone clinic cannot prescribe methadone to an opiate using patient from a doctor's office, the patient can get trapped in between and find no place to turn for pain relief. The problem is the methadone clinic treats substance abuse disorder and the pain doctor treats pain, and for now the two do not mix. As mentioned before if there was a 3rd option that allowed opiate dependent patients to be treated for pain, possibly with methadone, then this may be a better option for such patients who are chemically dependent on opiates strictly due to pain. However, at the time of this book, no such treatment actually exists, at least to my knowledge. And, if such a clinic is available, it might require a patient to relocate.

An Overview of Methadone Treatment

When a patient enters treatment they're usually started off on a low dose of methadone. The reason a low dose is prescribed, is because the doctor who prescribes the methadone is not completely sure what drugs a new patient has recently taken. A new patient might say they haven't used in 2 days when in truth they shot up an hour ago. To be medically safe, a doctor will prescribe a low dose of methadone. In many states the maximum intake dose is 30 mgs of methadone. Below is a diagram of a new patient getting a low dose of methadone.

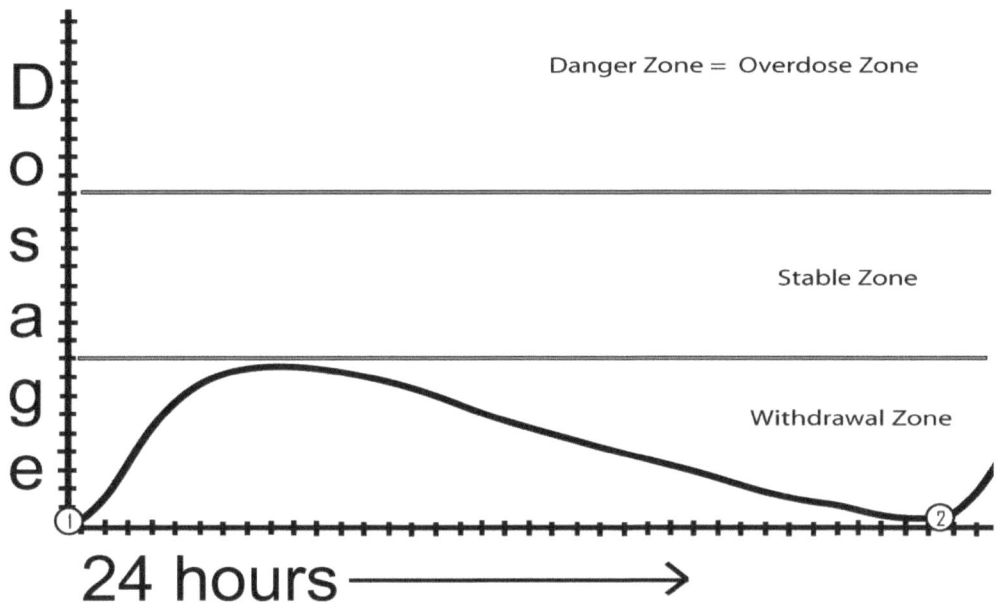

At point 1, when a patient takes their dose of methadone, the methadone begins to be absorbed into the bloodstream. The level of methadone in the body increases, and after about 3 hours the dose level in the blood reaches its peak. It is during the peak that a patient receives the greatest effect from the methadone in the form of reduced withdrawal symptoms and a reduction in cravings.

The liver begins to break down and metabolize the methadone, and the amount of methadone in the blood slowly decreases. The liver metabolizes 100% of the methadone in approximately 24 to 26 hours. Using the above diagram, you'll see that this patient's dose peaked in about 3 hours; however this patient remained in the Withdrawal Zone throughout the 24 hour period. This means these patient experienced withdrawals throughout their first day of treatment.

COMMON WITHDRAWAL SYMPTOMS INCLUDE: restless legs, tiny pupils (sometimes called pinned pupils), stomach ache, body aches, insomnia, irritability, loss of appetite, nausea, sweats, yawning, goose bumps, hot and/or cold flashes, and night sweats or heavy sweats.

As the liver metabolizes the methadone it is rendered harmless and is removed from the body in the urine and feces.

Methadone acts upon the opiate receptors slowly. Even though methadone is a thin watery liquid, I describe it as acting like molasses. Methadone moves slowly in the brain, delivers a light opiate effect (unlike heroin and other opiates that deliver a powerful opiate affect) and then the liver metabolizes the methadone slowly, again like molasses. Heroin and other opiates however move onto the opiate receptors very quickly, and deliver an explosion of opiate agonist activity, and then the liver breaks it down very quickly, and the "high" rapidly dissipates.

Because methadone produces the opiate effect (commonly called opiate agonist effect) that lasts for about 24 hours it makes for a great drug to help an opiate dependent brain get some opiate activity for an extended amount of time. Even though methadone opiate activity is small compared to heroin, morphine, and other opiates, its opiate agonist activity should last all day and all night when the dose level is correct.

It is important that a new patient return to the clinic the next day and request a dose increase. The nurses at the dosing window will ask a new patient how the methadone worked for them. They might ask,"How long did the methadone hold you?" Or they might ask, "How long did the methadone give you coverage." A new patient might answer, "I only got about 3 hours of coverage." The nurses will then ask about the withdrawal symptoms that were experienced by the patient and then they will write up an order (or type it into the computer) for a dose increase. All dose increases or decreases must be signed off by the doctor. In most clinics the turnaround for medical orders is 24 to 48 hours. This means that a new patient may have to take the same low dose of methadone again the second day in treatment, which means he/she will likely have another bad day, but not as bad a yesterday. Hey, nobody said that recovery is easy. Over the next several days a new patient should receive increasing doses of methadone, and as the doses increase the patient will feel better as they experience longer hours of "coverage."

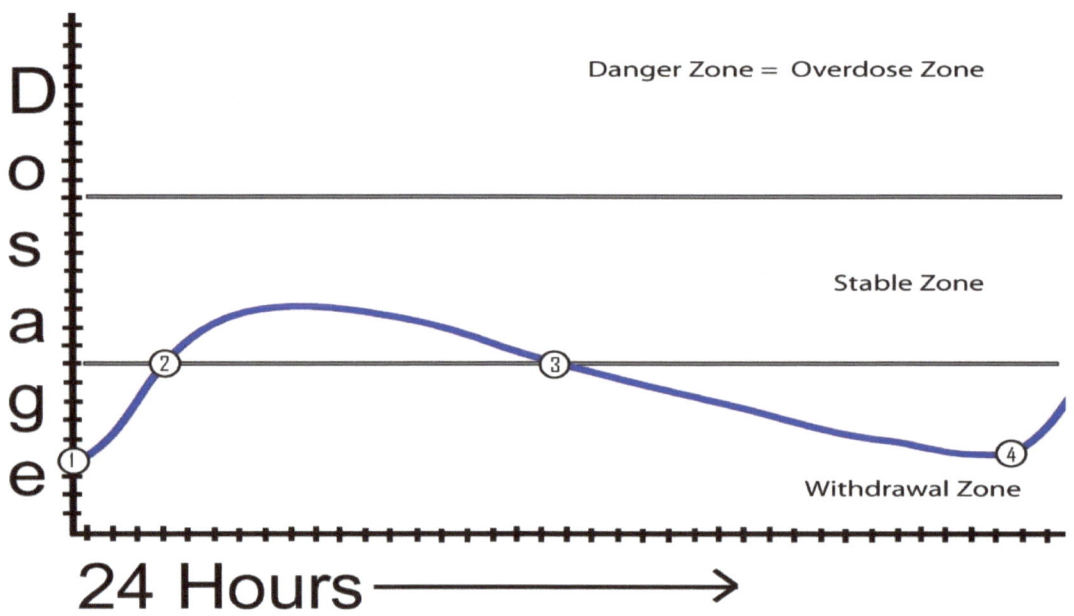

In the above example, this patient has received a dose increase. You'll see that this patient took their dose at point 1, and as the methadone entered the bloodstream this patient experienced some relief from withdrawals at point 2. From point 2 to point 3 this patient felt pretty normal. During this time frame this patient did not feel withdrawals or any *high* from the methadone. For many long time chemically dependent patients this time period is the first hour or 2 they've felt "normal" in years.

At point 3 however, the liver has diminished the amount of active methadone in the body to the point that withdrawal symptoms come back into play. This patient felt withdrawal symptoms for the remainder of their day. At point 4, they returned to the clinic the next day and took their next dose.

This patient is current in what we call the "induction phase" of treatment. During this phase of treatment the patient, the counselor, the nurses, and the doctor are all working to help this patient remain in treatment and find their therapeutic dose level, also known as their stable dose level. Since, patients are not getting a full 24 hours of relief from their withdrawals symptoms early in their treatment, many patient leave.

Unfortunately, many patients think that methadone will eliminate their withdrawal pains the first day. Sadly, this is usually not the case. I tell my client's they need to "fight for it if they seriously want to get clean."

After about 14 days most clients find their stable dose level. See the diagram below.

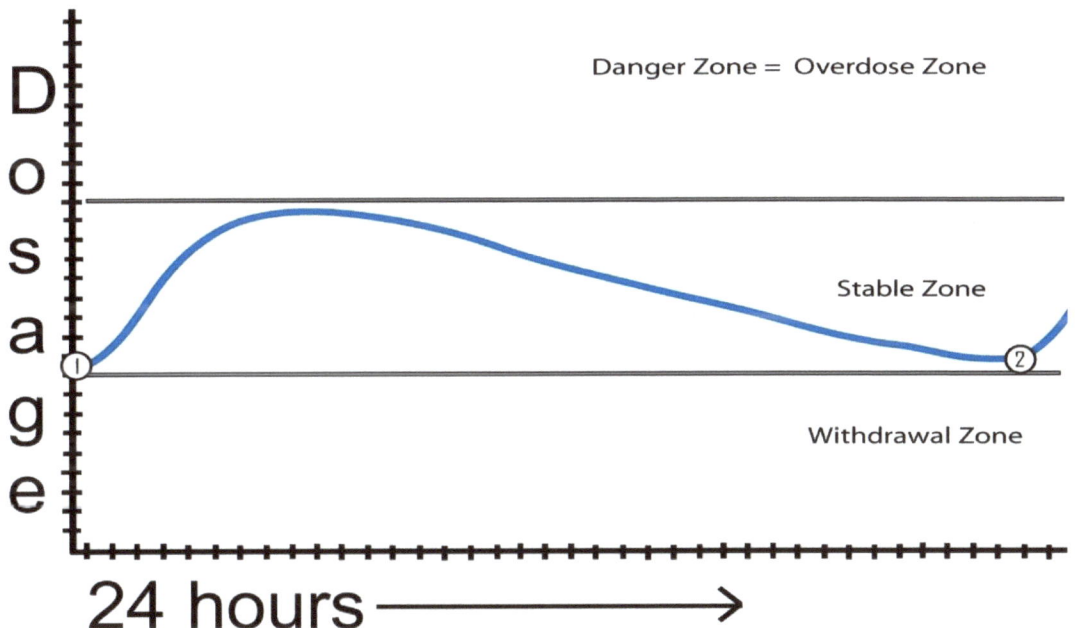

You'll notice that this patient received their dose at point 1, and when their methadone peaked after 3 hours they were still inside the "Stable Zone." As the methadone began to be metabolized by the liver the methadone in the body started to diminish, and after 24 hours this patient returned to the clinic for another dose. However, this patient remained in the Stable Zone throughout the 24 hour period. This patient never got high and never experienced any withdrawals. This patient is "in the pocket." This patient is at their stable dose level.

It is at this time that most of my patients tell me they haven't felt this good in a long time. I had one patient open up his wallet and show me a $20 bill. He said, "Look I actually have some money in my wallet, I'm gonna take my kids out to lunch for the first time in a year - normally I'd be out chasing pills with this money."

Some clients however at this point get depressed. They're stable, but they're not getting high. Many believe that methadone will get them high, and they want the high. Unfortunately, methadone moves too slowly to get someone high. Heroin and other opiates move into the blood and to the brain very quickly, and deliver an atomic bomb like explosion of opiate activity.

Methadone however, moves in slowly and only delivers a little tickle of activity.

Patients who keep "chasing the high" with methadone, soon find out that methadone just makes them sleepy, not high, when they take too much. Note that the goal of methadone treatment is not to get high, but to get stable. However many patients never seem to get this message and when they realize they are not going to get high from methadone, they start to slip and use street drugs. Often times we lose them as they slide. See the diagram below.

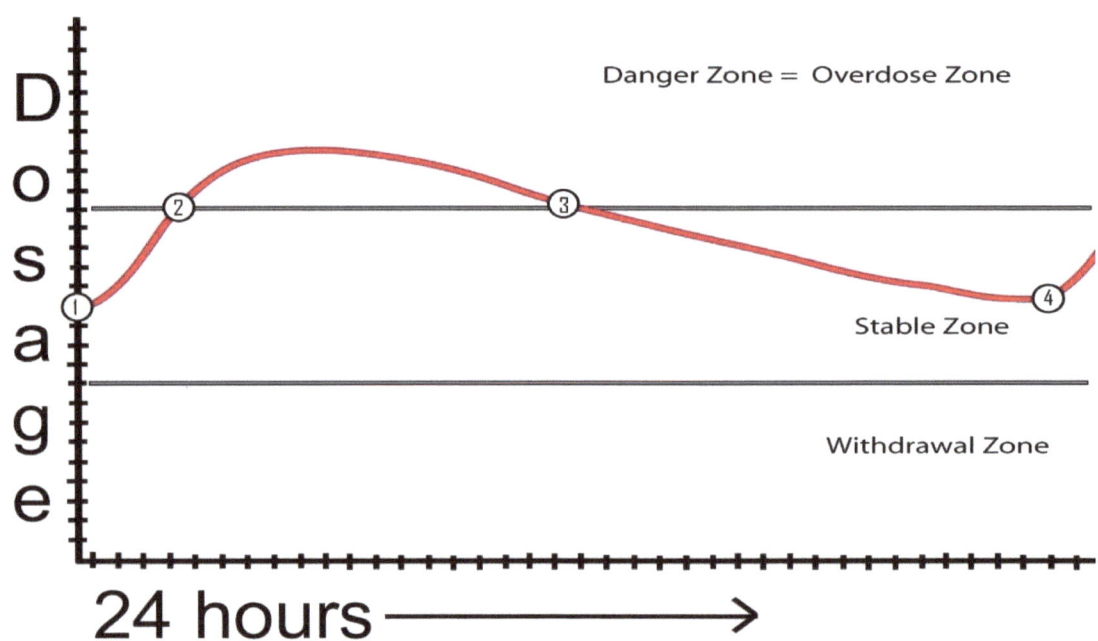

This patient took their daily dose at point 1. At point 2 this patient entered into the "Danger Zone/Overdose Zone." From point 2 to point 3 this patient likely got sleepy. Once the liver metabolized more of the methadone, this patient's methadone level fell back into the "Stable Zone" at point 3. Between points 3 and point 4 this patient was back to their normal-stable self.

Most patients at this point voluntarily ask for a dose decrease, and return to their stable dose level.

It is important to know that mixing methadone with other opiates can be dangerous, and can lead to an overdose. Although methadone blocks other opiates from attaching to the opiate receptors, methadone cannot stop "all" opiates from finding an open receptor. If an excessive amount of opiates are taken, it can lead to an overdose, even with methadones blocking ability. Methadone can be overpowered if enough opiates are taken.

The Triangle of Danger

Other drugs can also be dangerous when taken with methadone. Alcohol mixed with opiates (including Methadone and Buprenorphine), can be deadly. Opiates added to a benzo (benzodiazepines) can also be deadly. Benzodiazepines, as mentioned before include: Alprazolam (Xanax), Diazepam (Valium), Clonazepam (Klonopin), Lorazepam (Ativan), and others. See the "Triangle of Danger" below.

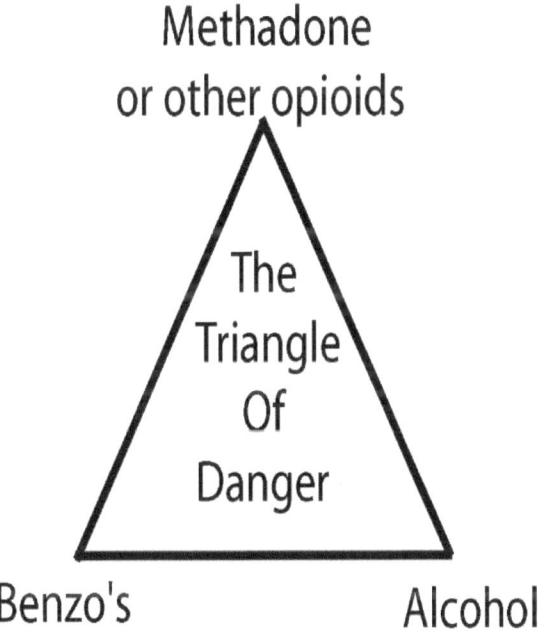

If you mix any two of these drugs you are at risk of dying. If you mix three of these drug types you are insane, and at risk of dying.

Healing The Brain

Whenever the brain is forced to accelerate the production of neuro chemicals above and beyond what is normal, it fatigues the brain. Much like a driver who spins his wheels, which does not move the car forward very much, it creates a lot of noise and smoke. The tires also wear out quicker. A brain that is repeatedly forced into overdrive also wears out prematurely. A chemically dependent brain lives as a slave to the master drug which regulates neurotransmitter production.

In most cases, illicit drugs don't directly make people high. Instead these drugs stimulate the brain to manufacture neurochemicals that the brain normally produces on its own. Normal day to day living however only demands a small amount of these neurochemicals. Illicit drugs however, trick the brain into making these pleasure and pain relieving neurochemicals in high volume, and command the brain to do so immediately.

The normal brain manufactures neurochemicals like Dopamine, Serotonin, Gaba, Acetylcholine, and others on its own. However, when the brain realizes its swimming in a sea of neurochemicals, often enough for 10 people, it naturally stops making more. The chemically dependent brain however, has been whipped into being a high volume chemical factory, driving euphoria, pleasure, and pain relief. The drug is the master and the brain is the slave. Over a period of time the brain no longer functions without the help of the master drug.

"Tolerance" is word used to describe how the drug loses its power over the brain, and the user is required to take more and more of the drug to get the same euphoric and pain relieving effects. The brain knows it's in trouble with the master drug, and as a self defense measure it closes some its neurochemical receptors. As more and more of these receptors close their doors, the user takes more and more drugs to drive the high volume demand thru the reduced number of receptors that are still open. It becomes a race between the closing of receptors and the delivery of more drugs to the open receptors, before the remaining open receptors also close their doors.

Eventually, the high can no longer be achieved because there are too few open receptors available. The brain is left with more closed receptors than open receptors. A brain with too few open receptors cannot get high, and the brain is in withdrawal. After all there are a limited number of receptors to process these neurochemicals. High-tolerance users usually continue to take drugs however, but their motivation is not to get high but rather to hold off withdrawals - but it's a zero sum game.

A normally functioning brain needs these neurochemicals in order to survive and function. However, when the addicted brain has to "wake up" and make these neurochemicals on its own, it becomes a painful and difficult task. This is what is known as withdrawals.

The truth is an addicted brain needs rest, and time to heal. The closed receptors need to come back online and open up again, however it is a painful healing process.

A rapid detox forces the brain into withdrawals and it is a form of brain trauma. It is a form of injury.

The brain needs time to re-learn how and when to manufacture these neurochemicals on its own.

Just as a person with a broken leg experiences pain while the bone heals, the body also experiences pain while the brain heals. A person with a broken leg needs crutches or a wheelchair to function normally, or nearly normal. An opiate damaged brain needs methadone. Methadone is the crutch or the wheel chair for the brain.

It is important to understand that the brain can function normally or nearly normal while on methadone. With methadone support, withdrawals are not a problem, and neither are cravings. Once a person gets stable on methadone, they can taper their doses down slowly, allowing the brain to heal slowly, while minimizing withdrawals along the way. This is just like a broken leg. When the bone begins to heal, it can slowly bear more weight, relying less on the crutch until the bone fully heals.

However, the brain itself is not the whole story. During recovery, a chemically dependent person also needs to get their life back on track. This is where counseling comes into play.

The Psychosocial Aspect of Recovery

In the counseling world we use the term "psychosocial." "Psycho" meaning the mind, and "social" meaning a person's interaction and functioning within society. The goal of counseling is to help a person fix their life problems so they can re-enter the straight world, become a functional member of humanity, and be a positive contributor to their family support system. The psychosocial aspect of a person's life is critical to achieve "full recovery."

Common psychosocial aspects of recovery can include:

1) **FAMILY** – this often includes children, parents, and other important people in a person's life. Many parents no longer trust their drug addicted child. Many patients recognize that their own addiction is hurting their marriage and their children. Many children are traumatized by the yelling and fighting associated with chasing pills and other drugs. These incidents create PTSD (Post Traumatic Stress Syndrome) in their children. Children who experience neglect or witness frightening events in the home often develop behavioral problems including fighting, anti-social behavior, inability to sleep, inability to concentrate, learning disabilities, and a disrespect for authority. Methadone allows a person to gain control

of their life, so they can manage a household and give time, love, and support to their children.

2) **HOUSING** is also a problem for many drug addicts entering into treatment. Some couples enter into treatment and have no money after years of chasing drugs. So they move in with Grandma and/or Grandpa along with their children. Living under the roof of a person means everyone has to live by the rules of the house. Many parents (Grandparents) do not trust methadone and do not approve of it. Most people who have never done drugs take the attitude, "Why don't you just quit?" This adds psychological hardship for those couples trying to recover from years of drug abuse. Many recovering couples learn that methadone gives them the relief they've searched for after many years of heavy drug use, only to endure ridicule and disapproval by their parents as they try to recover. This often leads many couples to abandon methadone treatment and relapse.

3) **LEGAL** problems often follow a recovering addict. Many are on parole and have to report to a parole officer. Others have upcoming court cases and face serious charges. All of this stress is compounded when children are involved. Many are under the scrutiny of DSS (Department of Social Services). The fear of incarceration by one or both parents puts additional strain on those who are new to recovery.

4) **MEDICAL** problems can also be a source of stress. Many drug addicts have HIV or a fear of having HIV. Many have Hep-C or a fear of having Hep-C. Many will try and avoid seeing a doctor for fear of what they might learn. I have seen others who wanted to address these issues immediately. Other medical issues can include diabetes, high blood pressure, liver disease, injuries, arthritis, digestive disorders, and pregnancy. These and other medical challenges need to be addressed by the patient, the counselor, and the medical staff at the clinic. Many clients need to be referred to a primary care physician depending on the nature of the illness. Clients often need the help of free or low costs clinics. Many clients new to treatment have severe dental problems. Those with unsightly teeth are often reclusive. Limited socialization is not good for self esteem or mental health. Many clients' have mental health conditions such as anxiety, obsessive compulsive disorders, and PTSD to name a few. These problems can often complicate recovery as well.

5) **EMPLOYMENT** is another big problem for those in recovery. Once a client gets stable on the methadone, they need to seek employment. Many have been chasing pills for years and have little or no job skills. Many do not know how to operate a computer in order to conduct a job search. Many do not have good job prospects. Those who do find employment often only find low wage jobs. A good counselor will help a patient find employment, by helping with a resume and looking online for job opportunities. However, a counselor usually has 50 or more clients and cannot devote an excessive amount of time in this area.

5) **TRANSPORTATION** is another common problem faced by those in recovery. There is the need to get to work every day, and there is also a need to commute to the methadone clinic

every day. Many clients live 20 to 40 miles from their clinic. A two way trip can be expensive. Many clients drive with expired tags and expired driver's licenses. Many clients do not own cars that are in good shape, and as such are always scrambling for tires, parts, and various repairs. Many clients bum rides with others in treatment. The cost of automobile repairs and gas can prevent many clients from making it to the clinic on a daily basis; and missing days at the clinic often leads to a relapse.

6) **SOCIAL and PEER GROUP** problems also need to be addressed. A peer group of drug addicted associates is a problem. A recovering addict has to find a way to say "no" to drugs and to the people who are not yet ready to seek recovery. Often time's one spouse is ready for treatment and the other is not. Other family members as well can be triggers for a relapse. A recovering addict needs to determine which people to let go of and which people to keep. This is not always an easy decision.

PSYCHOSOCIAL SUMMARY - The list above is just a basic list, and certainly does not cover all of the psychosocial challenges a person must manage in order to function productively in society. Consider also that some problems link together to form a chain of troubled issues that must be addressed. As an example many people have a need for child care, which could free a person up to interview for jobs, assuming they have the transportation to get to the interview. Such a person presumably needs computer skills to search for work, and an email address and a phone number. All of this is predicated on a person being able to read and write the native language. A person needs clothes for an interview as well as basic hygiene. When multiple problems are linked together it is extremely difficult to develop a single-shot solution. Life is a hard enough challenge for most folks as it is, however life is even more problematic when you add in the setbacks associated with substance abuse.

Time in Treatment

You might wonder at this point, how long someone needs to remain stable on methadone before they complete their treatment. The simple answer is – it depends on the person and their situation.

Many factors influence a person's "time in treatment." Many people, who ask me about methadone treatment, seem to think that a person's time in treatment is determined by how much street drugs a patient took. The truth is the quantity of street drugs a person has taken before entering treatment is *not* an indicator of how long someone should remain in treatment.

The actual quantity of drugs taken over the years has more of an impact on a person's income, living arrangements, job opportunities, job skills, education, and health than anything else.

Methadone treatment will get a long-time opiate abuser stable, but work needs to be done on the part of the patient to get their "life" stable as well. In order for a chemically dependent person to get their life stable, they usually need help from their counselor, family, employer, and other supports.

In the beginning of treatment, a patient's counselor will complete a "psychosocial," which is an exploration and documentation of a client's history. Some of the questions asked include whether or not a patient has ever been in substance abuse treatment before, are they employed, are they married or ever been married, do they have children, what is their education level, are there any legal entanglements this patient needs to address, what is the patient's living arrangements, what is the patient's medical status, and is this client considering suicide at this time.

Counselor also asks patients what their needs are. Many patients' need to get a job, while many others need to get their GED, learn how to use computers, while others need transportation, a place to live, and a doctor. Every patient has different needs outside of the obvious need to quit the use of illicit drugs.

So, getting back to the question of how long a person needs to be in treatment, let's examine a brief psychosocial profile of some patients. I want you the reader, to try and figure out which of the following patients need to be in treatment longer than the others. Also, if you can, predict which patients will likely exit treatment too early and relapse.

1) 19 year old female – unemployed – never married - addicted to Oxycodone for 4 years – recently delivered a baby which was given to DSS (Department of Social Services) until such time as DSS deems the mother worthy of taking responsibility for the newborn. This patient admitted she got pregnant at 16 and gave the baby to the father who was 18 at the time and lived with his mother. He too was drug addicted. She attempted suicide soon after her first baby was born, however she is devoted to her new baby and she has a new boyfriend who is the father. He too comes to the clinic and has a low wage job. She is very immature.

2) 38 year old male – never married no children - unemployed but has worked as an auto mechanic – rotten teeth and self conscious about his teeth – often complains of pain with his teeth – does not have a car and takes the bus to the clinic – lives with his alcoholic mother – cannot operate a computer and does not have an email address – comes to the clinic in dirty clothes – always respectful and polite

3) 44 year old female – husband also in treatment at the clinic – they spent so much money on drugs they lost their house – moved into her father's house with her elderly father – the father lives in one bedroom, she and her husband live in one bedroom, while their two high school children (boy and a girl) share a bedroom – husband is in and out of work – she hasn't worked in 20 years – they cannot afford methadone for two and constantly borrow money from her father to make ends meet – father gives them grief for going to the methadone clinic, and doesn't understand why they can't just stop going and just tough it out – they have

borrowed money from their daughter who works after school in a fast food restaurant – they have used their daughters money to pay for their own methadone treatment – having not made car payments on their daughter car in a few months and the mother is afraid the bank will repossess the daughters car - the daughter pays half the car payment herself – the daughter unaware that her parent have not been making payments on the car

4) 30 year old male – picks up odd jobs but will not get a real job – cannot read – cannot operate a computer – spends all morning hanging out in the parking lot begging for money to pay for his methadone - client gets angry and threatens people when they ask for their money back after they lent it to him a few days ago and he cannot pay it back today - doesn't spend time with his counselor – no family support – does not have a stable place to live

5) 53 year old male – unemployed – has liver disease – former alcoholic – strong family support – collects social security benefits – meets with his counselor on a regular basis – a likeable personality

6) 62 year old female – long history of arrests and incarcerations – long time drug user – has Hep-C – been in methadone treatment for 19 years – strong family support – sweet grandmother like lady – very smart

7) 32 year old female – on her 2nd marriage to a man who is on disability and cannot work – she has a child from her first marriage and the father has custody of her child – she misses her child terribly and cries when she talks about her son - her work is never stable and any job she gets only last a few weeks – she and her husband live with her parents who took out a loan on their house to pay for her treatment - she is stable on methadone for 3 years – she attempted to exit methadone treatment to save money, but after 12 days she returned due to withdrawals – she has low self esteem, and a new DUI charge

8) 27 year old female – divorced – has a stable job that is demanding and does not pay well – she has custody of her two children – her ex-husband is unemployed, rarely pays child support – she cannot pay rent after she pays for methadone – she lives with her mother from time to time but her mother is an alcoholic – she runs late to the clinic most of the time because she has to take her 2 children to different day care centers – she is usually late to work – her car is not running well and she cannot afford to get it fixed -   drug screens are starting to show positive for opiates and benzo's – her behavior lately is moody and tense and she has also begun avoiding her counselor.

The point of the above exercise was for you to recognize that people's lives are complex, and being able to determine a person's time in treatment cannot be calculated. Life is an unfolding series of events that cannot be predicted. So which of the patient above will need to be in treatment longer than others is simply too difficult to determine in advance.

Phases of Treatment plus a Discussion of Relapse

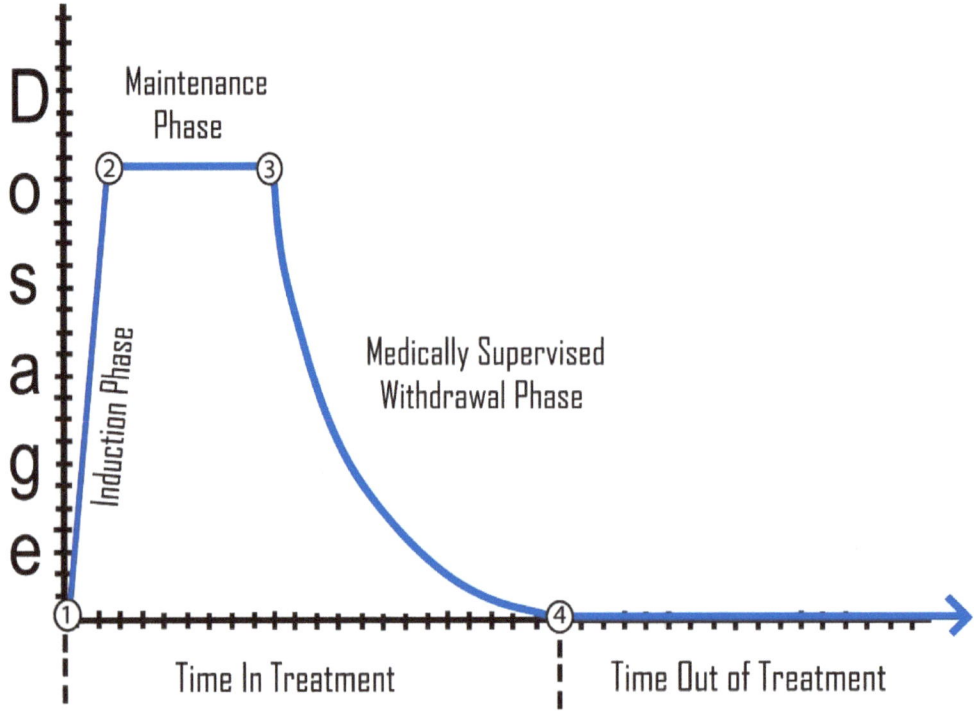

When a patient enters methadone treatment they're in what is called the "Induction Phase." During the Induction Phase a patient is not stable, as they have not yet found their therapeutic dose level. Patients in the Induction Phase should be monitoring their withdrawal symptoms and reporting their symptoms to their counselor as well as the nurses. They should also be receiving dose increases every few days as needed until they find their stable dose level. Once a patient finds they are receiving 24 hours of relief from withdrawals, as well as relief from cravings, they will have arrived at their therapeutic dose level.

I have seen many patients who refused to go above 100 mgs of methadone. I have concluded that somehow they have a psychological fear of going to a 3-digit dose level. I tell all my patients not to pay attention to the dose level, and instead pay attention to their withdrawal symptoms. Once they no longer have withdrawals for a full 24 hours they have probably found their stable dose level.

On the other side of the equation however are cravings. If a patient is otherwise stable, but has ongoing cravings they will likely benefit from a "slight" dose increase. A small dose increase at this point will usually eliminate cravings.

It is important to remind everyone that methadone is not a drug to get a patient high. The goal of methadone treatment is to get stable, not to get high.

Many patients quit methadone treatment because they never get high with methadone. Somehow many patients mistakenly think that methadone is supposed to get them high, much like the high they get from heroin or pain pills. This is not the way it works, and once *some* patients understand this, they start slipping, and revert back to taking illicit drugs. Soon these illicit drugs show up in their urine drug screens. Over time, patients who continue to turn in dirty drug screens, are eventually removed from the program. However, in truth, such patients tend to remove themselves from treatment. They usually just stop coming to the clinic and return to the street life.

Many however understand that turning back to street behaviors and illegal drug use is not a good option. Those with the right motivation understand their drug use affects their children, their family, their job, and their future. Patients with enough on the line will usually do what it takes to get clean, and rely on the methadone to hold back their withdrawals and their cravings, allowing them to move forward in life.

Once a patient finds their stable dose level and remains there for a long period they are said to be in the Maintenance Phase, also known as the Stabilization Phase. As a counselor, I tell my clients they should remain in the Maintenance Phase for a year, or two, or three. Many new patients, usually males, come into the clinic with what I call "male pattern thinking." I know this thinking well, as I too am a man.

Male thinking involves the use of cowboy logic, engineering, and a basic understanding of mechanics and electronics. They know they have a problem, and all they have to do is work the methadone tool to solve their problem and then move on to the next challenge. Unfortunately, addiction is not a quick fix.

Many young male clients come to me on their first day and say, "I'm only going to be here two weeks." I ask them, "Have you studied addiction?" Or I'll ask, "Have you ever read anything about methadone treatment?" And of course they have not, but even so, they are set in their ways and they stay two or three weeks and leave, only to return a month or two later with a new found respect for what it takes to get clean with methadone assistance.

The problem with these "short timers" is their expectations. They expect their addiction to be resolved in two or three weeks. They expect their strong will power to make them somehow stronger than the other people in the clinic. As if the other people in the clinic have weak willpower. It's a form of arrogance and ignorance. I often say, "A Navy Seal can't come off opiates without help, and Navy Seals are pretty tough aren't they?"

Below is graph of a patient who exits treatment during the Induction Phase (in red).

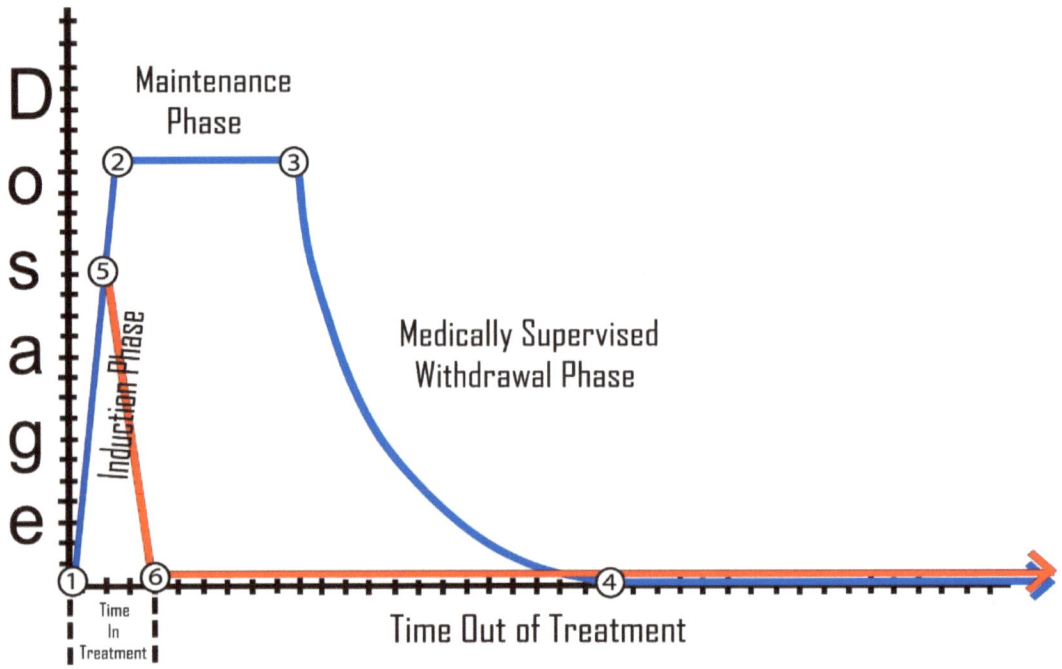

A committed patient will follow the blue line and progress thru points 1, 2, 3, 4 and exit treatment. A patient who follows the red line and follows points 1, 5, 6, 4 misses out on a lengthy time with counseling and an extensive loss of methadone support. The likelihood of a relapse for such a patient is extremely high.

Those who exit methadone treatment correctly stand the best opportunity to avoid a relapse. Many patients however, leave too soon, and their brain is not prepared to operate with an opiate deficit, and this leads to a relapse.

It's no wonder that those who leave treatment too early are ill prepared for the future; more often client's return to old habits, and relapse.

Now, imagine a client who chooses to leave treatment even before they reach their stable dose level. Such a treatment curve might look something like the following:

The goal of methadone treatment is to keep a person in the Stable Zone long enough for a person's brain to heal. A chemically dependent brain needs opiates to function without withdrawals. A person who lives with moderate to severe withdrawals is not able to work, manage a household, go to school, or otherwise pursue worthwhile productive activities.

So, while a person's brain gets stable with an opiate replacement (methadone), the patient also needs to stabilize the rest of their life. The Psychosocial aspects of their life that need to be stabilized can include: family relationships, support networks, financial problems, child care problems, legal problems, health problems, relationship problems, education problems, transportation problems, housing problems, and employment problems. Each of these areas needs to be fixed or at least addressed during the one, two, or three year Stabilization Phase.

Below is a graph of a patient who exits treatment once they reach the Maintenance Phase of treatment.

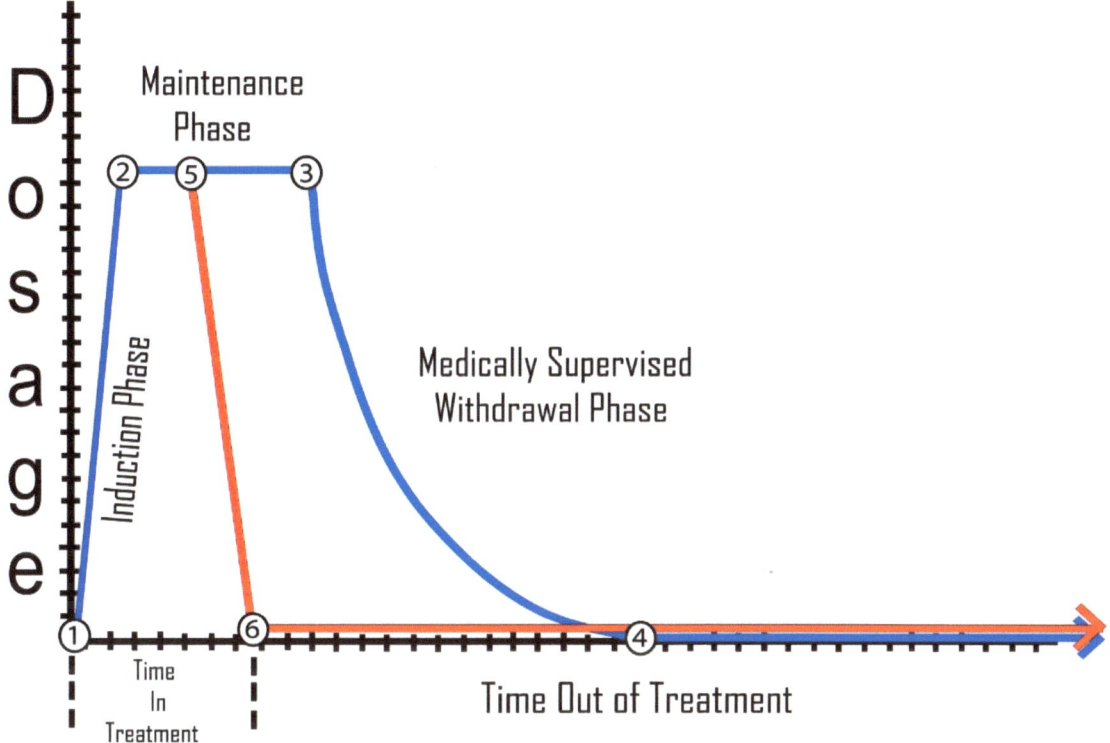

Again, imagine all the time lost for quality counseling support and opiate replacement therapy (methadone).

Assuming a patient remains in the Stable Zone for one, two, or three years they may find themselves ready to taper down their doses with an eye for exiting methadone treatment. Based on my personal observations as a methadone counselor, I've found that most patients who begin to taper down their doses need to be in the Medically Supervised Withdrawal Phase (MSW) for 9 months to a year or more.

I will admit that most patients do not spend enough time in the MSW Phase. Unfortunately, most get into such a hurry they exit treatment too soon. They often learn however that their organic brain is not able to give up its dependence on opiates quite as fast as their desire to leave methadone. The organic brain needs to heal slowly, and the patient is usually not willing to wait that long. As a result, many patients rush themselves out of treatment. See below:

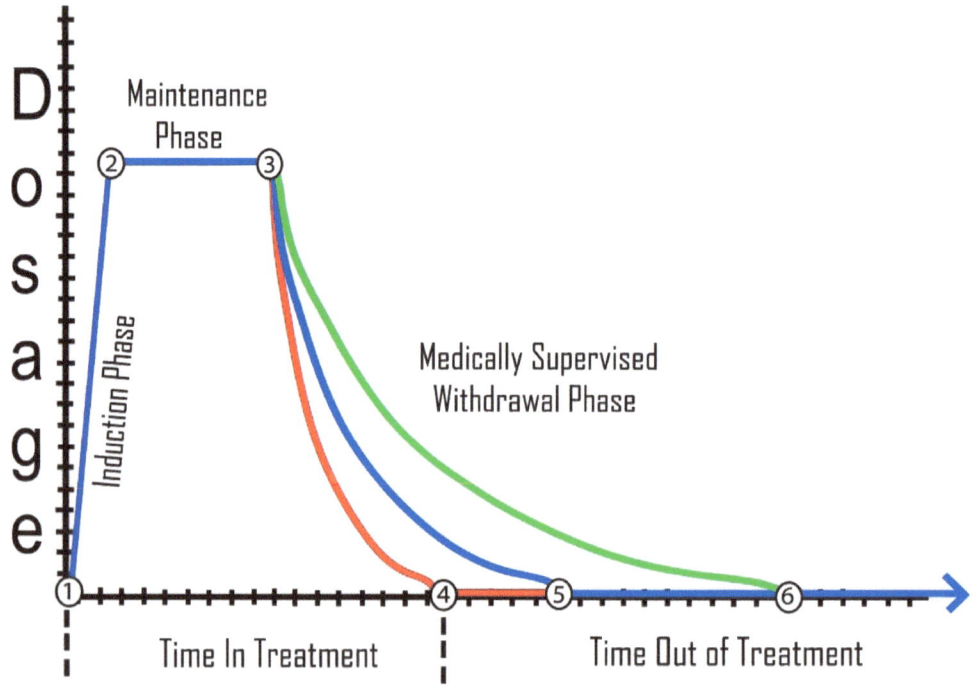

The red line follows a patient who exits the MSW Phase too early while a patient following the blue line has a better chance at long term recovery. A patient who follows a more extended MSW timeline, such as someone on the green line, has the best chance for long term sobriety.

Some patients are not honest with themselves and with the reality of their withdrawal symptoms. Instead many focus on reasons to exit treatment "now." In summary the best chances for a long term recovery and avoidance of a relapse is a lengthy amount of time in the Maintenance Phase, followed by an extensive amount of time in the MSW Phase. The brain needs time to heal, and the brain heals slowly.

I've known many patients use positive can-do language to convince themselves they can get off methadone by Christmas. Or they want to be out of treatment when their kids start school, or they want to be out of treatment this summer so they can take the kids on vacation. These are all well and good aspirations, however in many cases the "organic brain" is still dependent on opiates, and is not paying attention to the calendar or any vacation plans. The organic brain will heal as quickly as it can; and a person needs to give their brain the time it needs. The organic brain always seems to heal slower than what the patient want it to.

This is much like a person with broken leg who is in a hurry to remove their cast. Many people are known to remove a leg cast early, only to find their leg is not fully healed. The same is true with methadone patients who exit treatment too soon. Many find their brain is simply not ready yet, and return to the clinic and start over.

I've witnessed many of my patients drop down several milligrams of methadone and say to me, "You know I really don't feel that bad, I think I'll be out of here in a month." I caution my patients not to get cocky; and let their withdrawal symptoms tell them whether they are ready to come down another 10 milligrams or not. Most patients who "honestly" pay attention to their withdrawal symptoms, and use their withdrawal symptoms as their guide, are the ones who give the MSW Phase the ample time necessary to get clean and stay clean.

Model 1

Model 1 is the way most people think about methadone treatment. This is would include patients, parents, spouses, doctors, nurses, counselor, judges, police, school teachers, and just about everyone.

Model 1 proposes that a patient will enter into methadone treatment, get stable on methadone, exit methadone treatment correctly and then live the rest of their life drug free.

Many of my clients, when they consider Model 1, realize that once they leave treatment they are expected to live drug free for another 20, 30, 40, or even 50 years.

Below is a graphic of Model 1.

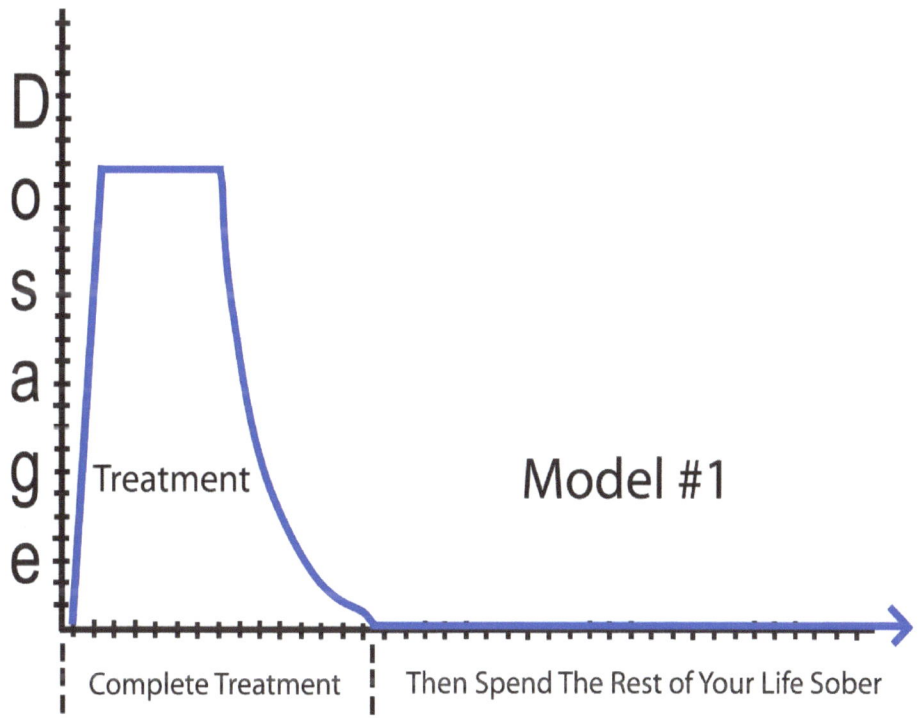

Consider the following:

National Institute on Drug Abuse - *"Addiction is defined as a chronic, relapsing brain disease that is characterized by compulsive drug seeking and use, despite harmful consequences."*

When I came across this definition, I was shocked by the words "chronic relapsing brain disease." Other words for "chronic" include: life-long, constant, unceasing, persistent, and never-ending. So, according to this modern definition of drug addiction, a person is going to have a lifetime of repeated relapse episodes.

When I first read this definition I thought, "*If* this definition is correct, and it's a big *if*, then Model 1 is incorrect, because Model 1 does not account for any relapses."

Consider the following "Relapse Model of Addiction."

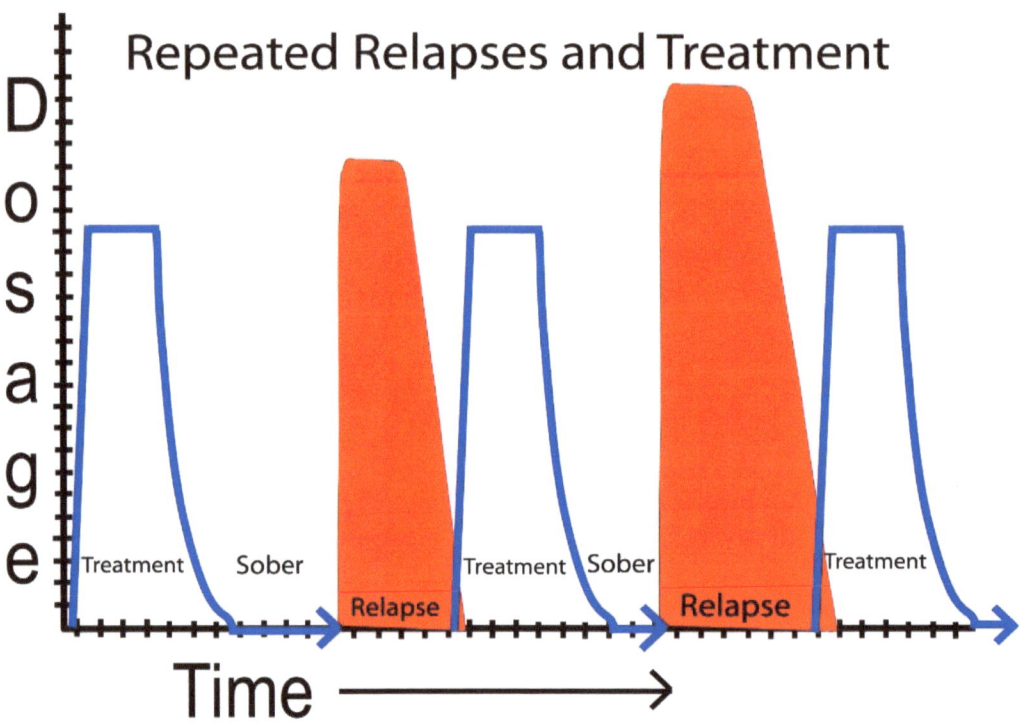

According to the Relapse Model of Addiction, a person enters treatment, gets sober for a period, and then relapses, only to re-enter treatment again, get sober again, and relapse again, only to continuously repeat the cycle.

When I show this graphic to my clients, many of them light up and say, "That's me, this is my third time here," or something similar.

I had one client tell me about a 9 month relapse episode in which he destroyed his marriage, lost custody of his kids, lost his house, sold his truck, maxed out his credit cards, and exhausted his savings, all in the pursuit of drugs.

Obviously, a relapse episode is a dangerous time period. I've heard countless stories of people who relapse and end up in some kind of deep trouble.

You'll notice that in the graphic above, that the second Relapse Period is larger than the first. This is because most of my clients have told me that each relapse is worse than the one before.

Due to this understanding of addiction, I felt compelled to find a better solution. I eventually came up with what I call Model 2. See below:

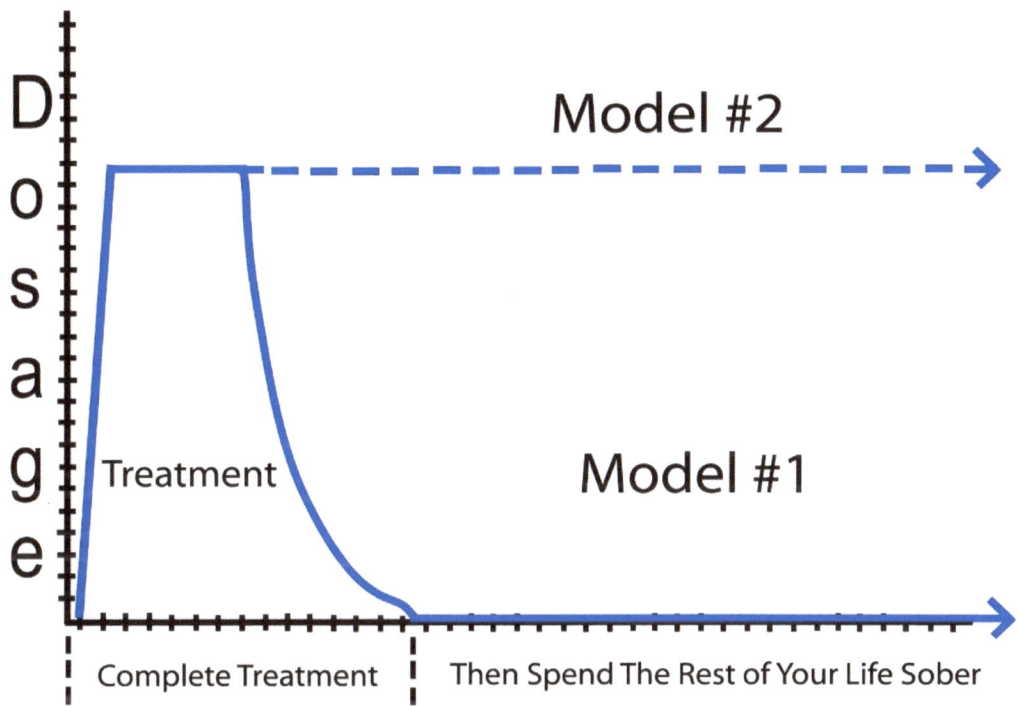

As you can see we have Model 1, with Model 2 represented by the broken lines.

The concept of Model 2 is that a person can avoid the Relapse Model of Addiction by simply staying on methadone over the long run, therefore avoiding high risk relapses.

After all, methadone is a safe and legal drug that has been dispensed and studied since the 1960's. Studies have shown that those addicted to opiates, who take methadone correctly are less likely to commit crimes, less likely to be incarcerated, more likely to be employed or in school, and less likely to spread diseases like Hep-C and HIV through needle use.

In addition, studies have shown that those who are addicted to opiates and choose to participate in methadone treatment are more likely to re-establish employment and eliminate criminal activity.

I have a client who has been in methadone treatment for over 19 years, another 3 who have been in treatment for over 12 years, and several around the 8 year mark. I've heard of people who have been in methadone treatment for over 30 years. Some of my clients tell me that they are afraid to leave methadone treatment, because they know they will likely relapse.

Also, some have said that their family is afraid of what they might do if they leave methadone treatment. So, they just "cruise" through life on methadone and most of their friends, family, and coworkers are none the wiser.

You might be surprised to learn that some of the people you know, and like, are in methadone treatment.

The Prevailing Attitude Regarding Methadone Treatment

Most people these days seem to have a dim view of methadone treatment. And, many point to studies and statistics that put methadone treatment in a bad light. There are statistics that I have seen that show that only 2% of patients who exit methadone treatment are drug free after 10 years of sobriety.

Such a statistic makes methadone look pretty bad. However this is based on Model 1.

It would appear to me that if 2% of the people who exited methadone treatment were drug free for 10 years, the other 98% of the people must have either followed the Relapse Model, or died. Such a study would not account for those who followed Model 2, because they remained in treatment.

Studies do support what has already been presented earlier, that people who are addicted to opiates and choose to participate in methadone treatment are less likely to get into trouble with the law and more likely to be productive and contribute to their family.

I propose that if the world looked at methadone treatment, and focused on those who remain on Model 2, rather than focus on Model 1 and the Relapse Model; then methadone would look to be a much stronger alternative for those who are currently addicted opiates. The benefits of Model 2 would also carry into society the likelihood of less crime with less police action, less disease with lower health care costs, and an increase in taxes being paid by those who are re-employed due to their lives now being stable. Those who are re-employed will also contribute to the local economy with everyday purchases of food, clothing, shelter, and consumer goods, rather than rely on food stamps and other government assistance. Children would also be released from DSS (Department of Social Services) to the custody of their natural parents since their parents are no longer involved with illegal drugs and criminal activity.

A New Look At Opiate Addiction as a Disease

There are many models of addiction and one is known as the "disease model." My company embraces the disease model. Today many people still hold fast to the concept of Model 1, which implies that the disease of opiate addiction can be cured. However, many believe that addiction cannot be cured; only treated. I often tell my clients that methadone treatment is just that, a treatment, not a cure.

When patient's relapse, they often blame methadone and the clinic. I say, "Don't blame the methadone, blame the opiate addiction," after all which came first? After all, what is methadone treating in the first place?

The disease model of addiction does not necessarily imply that there is a cure. There are many diseases for which modern science does not have cure.

Model 1 treats the disease of addiction like a broken leg or an infection, which is actually an injury or a condition, not a true disease. A broken leg does follow Model 1, in that it can be put in a cast, the bones can heal, and the leg is as good a new. As with an infection, such as an ear infection, an antibiotic kills the invading bacteria and the person is cured. However, such is not the case as of yet for the disease of opiate addiction.

Addiction is a disease much like diabetes or hypertension. With diabetes there is no cure, however it can be managed. It is true that managing diabetes involves the hassle of finger sticks and blood sugar readings; but the disease can often be well controlled with medication, like insulin. Those with diabetes understand that it is a lifelong condition, because as of yet there is no cure. Hypertension is not always curable either, but it can often be managed with medication and lifestyle changes. Hypertension, like diabetes is a lifelong medical challenge. The disease of opiate addiction is also a controllable disease, with use of methadone or Buprenorphine as the primary medications, and in the opinion of many it is also a lifelong condition.

Positron emission tomography, better known as a PET Scan, is a brain imaging technology that measures the glucose metabolism of tissues and cells in the body. PET Scans of addicted individuals show a reduced level of glucose metabolism in various regions of the brain. This particular pattern is common to most addicted individuals, regardless of which drug was the drug of choice. As an addicted individual recovers from their addiction however, their brain centers show an improvement in brain function, as evidenced by increasing glucose uptake. Unfortunately however, these regions never quite recover to the level of a never-addicted brain. Is this why chemically dependent people relapse? The answer is unclear. This evidence does indicate however, that the brain has undergone permanent changes.

I have some say to me, "Yea, well maybe addiction is a disease, but people choose to use drugs and so they brought the disease upon themselves." My response is, "Well you may be right, however many people with diabetes and heart disease may have brought it upon themselves as well, by choosing unhealthy diets, smoking cigarettes, and avoiding exercise; but we still treat those people, right?."

Methadone Is Just A Substitute for Heroin

I hear many people tell me that methadone is just a substitute for heroin. Is it?

Let's look at a 24 to 48 hour heroin curve below:

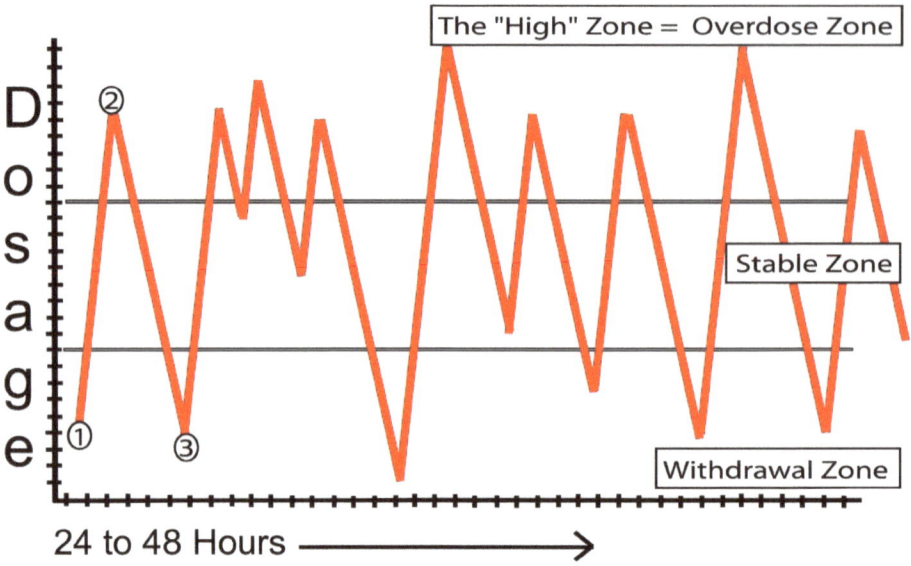

At point 1 on the graph above is when a heroin user wakes up in the morning and gets their first fix, whether it be by injecting or by smoking heroin. As you will see, the "high" or the "rush" comes on very quickly. That's because opiates like heroin, when injected, is undiluted and bypasses the liver, which allows it to travel straight to the brain. Once undiluted heroin is in the brain it attaches to the available opiate receptors where it delivers a powerful blast of opiate activity, also known as opiate agonist activity. If the heroin or opiate pills were to be taken orally, they would make their way to the liver where they would be metabolized to some degree, and then move on to the brain. Due to the metabolic activity of liver, the opiate would be somewhat diminished in strength once it reaches the brain. This is why many users often turn to needle use.

In the example above, at point 1 the user gets their first fix, and as you can see the opiate activity ramps up very quickly because the opiate is bypassing the liver, and once in the brain it delivers a blast of opiate agonist activity. However, heroin and other opiates give up the goods very quickly. They are short lived opiates. Once their opiate agonist delivery is complete, they are ejected from the opiate receptors and find their way back to the circulatory system, where they are eventually removed from the body.

As you can see, the opiate agonist activity peaks very quickly at point 2. This usually occurs after a few seconds. The high tends to last 5 to 10 minutes before it starts to fade. As the high is degraded, if the user does not find another fix soon they will quickly slide into the Withdrawal Zone. The feeling of withdrawal is a powerful motivator to find another fix. For most long term users, the fear of withdrawals is more powerful than the thrill of the high, *and most report that there is no high anymore.*

When opiate activity reaches its peak, this can be the moment when some people die as a result of an overwhelming delivery of opiate agonist activity. This is generally referred to as an "overdose."

All day long a heroin user is motivated to stay out of the Withdrawal Zone. So as soon as the high fades, it's a scramble to find more money to buy the next fix. As the high retreats, the user begins a desperate search for money, and at this point, an addict will do desperate things, including illegal activities. These activities are generally referred to as "drug seeking activities," or "drug seeking behaviors."

For someone who is opiate dependent, once they start coming down from the high, they go into *money seeking mode*. Once the money is acquired they go into *drug search mode*. Once the drug is located they often must travel to get their drug. Many will drive at high rates of speed. Many will take their children along with them to acquire their drugs. Once the drug is acquired, they go into *using mode*. And then the cycle repeats throughout the day, because the high doesn't last very long.

As you may remember, methadone does not fade very quickly. Methadone will deliver opiate agonist activity over a long period of time. Methadone will remain in the opiate receptors for several hours giving the user 24 hours worth of relief from withdrawals and cravings.

Now take another look at the Heroin Graph above. Try to imagine a person chasing heroin all day, and all night, and desperately trying to avoid withdrawals, and ask yourself, "Can that person hold a job?" and "Can that person raise a family?" The answer is probably "NO."

Now look at the graphic below of a stable methadone patient.

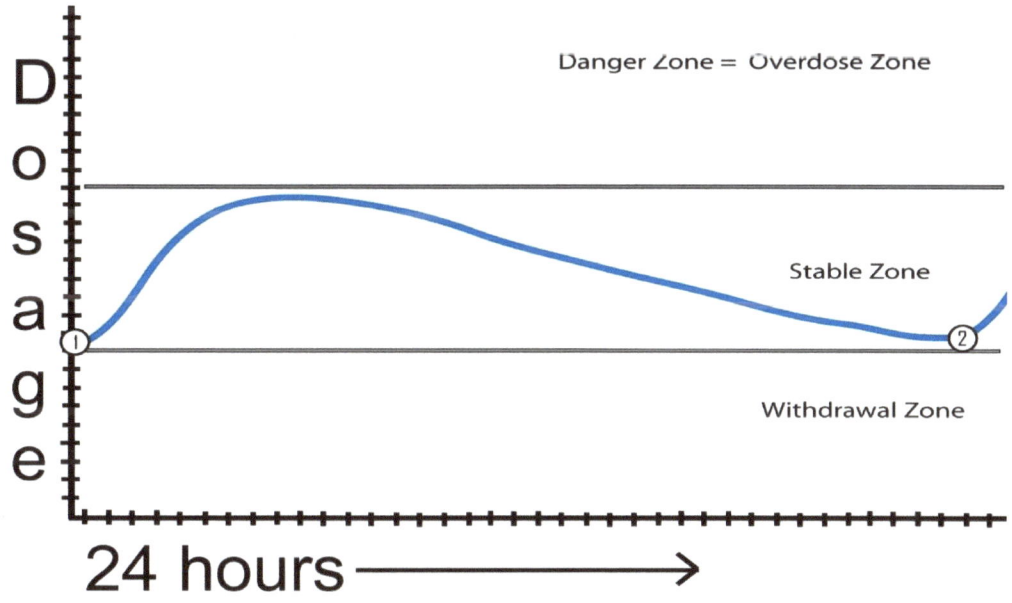

Ask yourself, "Can this person hold a job, raise a family, and go to school?" The answer is probably, "YES."

So is methadone treatment a substitute for heroin? I say, "No, it's a game changer."

Many clinics offer Buprenorphine as an alternative to methadone. Buprenorphine is a good drug. Many doctors are now dispensing Buprenorphine to clients, and many clients are able to receive a 30 day supply. A common problem with this type of arrangement is that many doctors do not provide adequate counseling. In addition, placing a 30 day supply of an addictive drug in the hands of an opiate dependent person often leads to abuse. Client's often think that if one pill works then two pills will work better. Soon many clients run out of pills in the middle of the month and start to use street drugs. At a clinic however, Buprenorphine as well as the methadone is dispensed and controlled by the clinic; so such abuses do not occur as often. Clients are able to earn take home doses however after they have proven worthy of the responsibility.

For unbiased information regarding the science of addiction and treatment let me suggest the following resources:

National Institute on Drug Abuse (NIDA) - https://www.drugabuse.gov/

Substance Abuse and Mental Health Services Administration (SAMSHA)

https://www.samhsa.gov/

National Institute on Alcohol Abuse and Alcoholism (NIAAA) |

https://www.niaaa.nih.gov/

Other publications by Travis Nevels and T3Publications.com:

Methadone and Pregnancy

Opiates, Methadone, and Detox